FIBROMYALGIA

A Guide to Understanding the Journey

By Shelly Bolton

New Dawn Publishers, 2013

Printed in the United States of America

Table of Contents

INTRODUCTION

Chances are- if you are reading this- you or someone you love has been diagnosed with fibromyalgia or suspects that it is present. Assuming that is the case, you are probably looking to answer some important questions:

* Do you really know what fibromyalgia is?

* If you do *not* have it but someone you *know* does: how much do you know about what they are going through?

* If *you* have it, or suspect that you do: how often do you feel as if you are all alone, and maybe crazy- or just imagining things- because there are no outward signs that would account for the pain you are feeling?

* How often does the idea "I'm too young to be falling apart!" cross your mind?

The causes for this disorder, as well as effective treatments or possible cures, are quite elusive. While doctors, as well as patients and their families, search for answers- something that seems to offer at least a bit of relief to sufferers is simply knowing that you are not alone, and that you are not crazy, but rather that the pain is caused by a very real condition. It can also be helpful for family members to understand a bit more about what the "fibromite" (a loving term coined by and used within the fibromyalgia community) is going through.

> ☺
>
> Yeah, yeah- I know those of you with fibro are now saying "Relief??? You call that relief???" Just know that although the relief you are really hoping for is physical, the emotional relief that comes from knowing you're not alone and having your family understand you better does make a difference.

With these ideas in mind I set out to find literature that might help illuminate the details of our struggle, but could not find any one source that I felt really clearly spelled out the daily issues with which I was dealing and explained them so that people on the outside could understand. So, I decided to put together my own resource using the information I could compile from several sources as well as incorporating my own story, and adding some details to help explain it in simple, everyday terms.

If you have fibromyalgia yourself, then much of this will likely resonate with you. I found it helpful to understand that the majority of the symptoms I experience are actually quite common for fibromites, and that there have actually been studies which provided scientific evidence that the pain and other symptoms experienced in fibromyalgia are quite real, rooted in the central nervous system[1] (and not imagined or "psychosomatic" as has been suggested in the past). If you have a loved one who has fibromyalgia, then chances are it frustrates you that you cannot even really understand what they are going through, let alone fix the problem. I cannot tell you how to fix it, but as you read through this guide you may have a 'lightbulb' moment- or two- in which you begin to understand some of the outward signs and behaviors of your loved one as *reactions* to what they are experiencing.

Now, you or your loved one most likely have an experience that is somewhat different from my own, and I am not going to try to write this as an "everyman," since there really is no such thing with fibro. Everyone's experience is unique, and since I have not had your experience, I must use my own. Please understand that some people experience associated conditions and symptoms that are not addressed here and that this is by no means an exhaustive source on the subject. Although the bulk of this writing involves the description of symptoms, related conditions, and their effects, this is not intended to be a checklist or a guide for diagnosis, but rather a guide to understanding from a personal and family-oriented perspective.

Although the journey is not one that a sane person would consider "enjoyable", I hope that you enjoy this guide in that it helps you to understand the condition a bit better. And maybe in understanding the condition, understand your loved one or yourself a bit more than before.

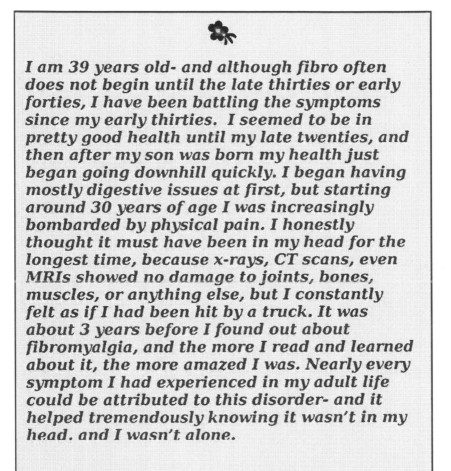

I am 39 years old- and although fibro often does not begin until the late thirties or early forties, I have been battling the symptoms since my early thirties. I seemed to be in pretty good health until my late twenties, and then after my son was born my health just began going downhill quickly. I began having mostly digestive issues at first, but starting around 30 years of age I was increasingly bombarded by physical pain. I honestly thought it must have been in my head for the longest time, because x-rays, CT scans, even MRIs showed no damage to joints, bones, muscles, or anything else, but I constantly felt as if I had been hit by a truck. It was about 3 years before I found out about fibromyalgia, and the more I read and learned about it, the more amazed I was. Nearly every symptom I had experienced in my adult life could be attributed to this disorder- and it helped tremendously knowing it wasn't in my head, and I wasn't alone.

GENERAL OVERVIEW

If you have gotten this far then you probably already know that fibromyalgia is a condition that involves widespread (sometimes severe) pain that is not otherwise explained. This condition and the associated pains are not caused by injury or other deformity or illness. Fibromyalgia does not refer to pain in general or a short term issue but rather a defined condition of chronic (long-term), widespread pain that occurs throughout the body.

The criteria used by the medical community to determine fibromyalgia include the occurrence of pain in all four quadrants of the body (left *and* right sides, above *and* below the waist) and the presence of at least 11 of 18 specific tender points in which pain occurs when light pressure is applied[2]. The criteria used by the American College of Rheumatology also include axial skeleton involvement[3], meaning that there would be at least some pain in the spine, skull, and/or rib cage[4]. The term "widespread" also indicates that the pain extends not only to all quadrants of the body, but also occurs in multiple areas and tissue types such as bone, joint, muscle, skin, etc. The pain of fibromyalgia is chronic, or long term, meaning that it lasts a minimum of 6 months[5] * (though for most fibromites this is a lifelong condition). There are many other symptoms which, though not necessary as diagnostic criteria, are often present alongside fibromyalgia. Many of these symptoms and associated conditions are something most "normal" people have experienced from time to time, but it is their frequency and severity that put them into the symptom or condition category.

One of the biggest issues fibromites face, other than pain, is fatigue. Fibromyalgia is, in fact, considered to be very closely related to CFS (Chronic Fatigue Syndrome)[6], and fatigue is one of the most common symptoms in fibro patients- occurring in over 80% of cases[7], and second only to pain. Even without any insomnia or other sleep disturbances, fibromites tend to overwhelmingly report pervasive fatigue that impairs their ability to participate in everyday activities.

In addition to general fatigue, a common symptom in fibromyalgia is an extreme reaction to physical exertion, often a bit delayed. This does not refer to the sore muscles that the average person experiences after exercise, but rather the achy, nauseated, dizzy, and sometimes feverish sensation that you would expect when you are coming down with the flu. It may not occur immediately after the physical exertion, but over the next several hours and sometimes into the next couple of days.

---

[*] some sources say 3 months
http://www.nlm.nih.gov/medlineplus/ency/article/000427.htm

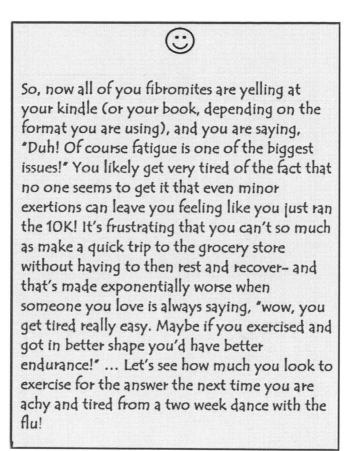

So, now all of you fibromites are yelling at your kindle (or your book, depending on the format you are using), and you are saying, "Duh! Of course fatigue is one of the biggest issues!" You likely get very tired of the fact that no one seems to get it that even minor exertions can leave you feeling like you just ran the 10K! It's frustrating that you can't so much as make a quick trip to the grocery store without having to then rest and recover- and that's made exponentially worse when someone you love is always saying, "wow, you get tired really easy. Maybe if you exercised and got in better shape you'd have better endurance!" ... Let's see how much you look to exercise for the answer the next time you are achy and tired from a two week dance with the flu!

Another delayed reaction seen in fibro patients is the response to stressful events, such as severe illness of a spouse or child, divorce, or loss of a loved one. As well as being delayed, these responses can be more physical in nature than one might expect. A common result of highly stressful events in a fibromyalgia patient might include the occurrence of extreme nausea and abdominal cramping, as well as reactions typically tied to an emotional event, such as panic attacks. In a fibro patient these reactions may not be seen until days or even weeks after the event.

Fibromites also are prone to hot flashes and night sweats -which, by the way, are not restricted to night time- similar to those that occur around the time of menopause. The biggest difference is that the fibromyalgia patient may be several years pre-menopause when this phenomenon begins, and it may continue for years- well into post-menopausal age. Many fibro patients describe feeling as if their body's thermostat is broken. This lack of proper temperature regulation in the body may be the result of irregular levels of certain neurotransmitters, including those that help regulate and maintain body temperature.

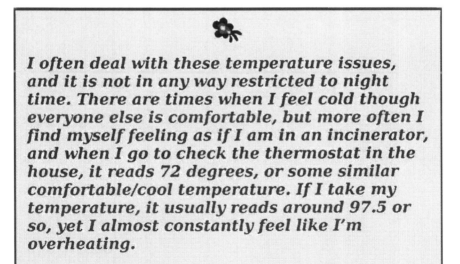

I often deal with these temperature issues, and it is not in any way restricted to night time. There are times when I feel cold though everyone else is comfortable, but more often I find myself feeling as if I am in an incinerator, and when I go to check the thermostat in the house, it reads 72 degrees, or some similar comfortable/cool temperature. If I take my temperature, it usually reads around 97.5 or so, yet I almost constantly feel like I'm overheating.

There are other general symptoms that occur with fibromyalgia, including frequent, severe migraine headaches. These headaches can occur from daily to a few times weekly, and are severe enough to be accompanied by visual disturbances and nausea. Sensitivity to light, sound, and smell are also common in fibro patients and can increase these headaches. The headaches that commonly occur with fibro can also play a big part in the concentration problems we will address later on.

MUSCLE/TISSUE RELATED SYMPTOMS

The primary earmark trait that is shared by all fibromyalgia patients and is the basis for diagnosis of this condition is widespread chronic pain. By widespread, it is meant that the pain is experienced in many areas of the body. If you think of the body in four quadrants, divided along the waist horizontally and along the vertical midline, pain that is truly "widespread" will occur in all four quadrants. It will at times be more severe in one area and less in another, but with fibromyalgia there will be chronic, recurring, often constant pain in all four quadrants.

There is no one type of pain that is "typical" for fibro patients. The pain from patient to patient, and even within the same patient, varies in type and intensity. There are three primary types of pain that are medically defined, including hyperalgesia and allodynia, which we will address in this section, and painful paresthesias, which you will find discussed in the section on neurological symptoms. However, there are other variations in pain type as well that have not been separated into medical categorizations. These are well described by author Adrienne Dellwo in her article on "Understanding Fibromyalgia Pain."[8] She describes a sudden stabbing pain, often in the chest or abdomen, which she labels "knife-in-the-voodoo-doll." This pain seems to come out of nowhere, and can be crippling. These stabs of pain in the soft tissues of the chest and abdomen can actually cause the patient to jump or become doubled over in the attempt to make the pain subside. Ms. Dellwo also describes a sensation that many people outside of fibro patients would not experience as pain, but which can become so pervasive in the case of fibromites that it can actually be painful. This she refers to as "rattled nerves," and it can be described as a sort of sensory overload, where certain sounds, smells, visual stimuli such as flashing lights or loud patterns, as well as other stressful situations can set the sufferer on edge. In addition to dizziness and a general anxiety, such occurrences can also cause nausea and even physical pain in the body of a person with fibromyalgia. When this type of pain is occurring, each sound, smell, movement, light, or other sensory stimulus can feel like a hammer to the head or body of the person experiencing the phenomenon.

Another associated condition that often occurs alongside fibromyalgia seems as if it would be related to the "knife-in-the-voodoo-doll" pain referred to previously, except that it affects the ribcage and cartilage instead of the soft tissues. It is actually a separate condition called costochondritis. This refers to a condition of swelling or inflammation of the cartilage at the junction of the ribs and sternum. When a flare-up occurs it results in severe chest pain that can mimic a heart attack. These occurrences can last from a few minutes to a few weeks and are often accompanied by soreness in and around the rib cage and a sharp increase in pain with coughing, sneezing or deep breaths. Although the relationship between costochondritis and fibromyalgia is unknown, it is reported in approximately 60-70% of fibro patients[9].

Of the medically defined types of pain that are common in fibromyalgia patients, hyperalgesia is perhaps the most common and has the widest definition. Rather than a specific sensation, this condition refers more to the intensity of pain. In fibromyalgia patients, the brain basically seems to amplify pain signals, causing them to be more severe than normal. This means that something that may cause mild to moderate pain in a "normal" person may cause pain that is moderate to severe in a fibromite. This also means that something that may not even cause perceivable pain in others can cause pain in fibro patients. Let's be clear, however, that this is not the same thing as a "low pain threshold," or "low pain tolerance," as understood by the layperson. That phrase implies that the person reacts more severely to the same level of pain, or simply isn't as strong-willed in tolerating pain. Hyperalgesia is a condition in which the actual pain level is higher than normal.

Allodynia[10] is a pain type that is most common to medical conditions such as peripheral neuropathy, but very rare outside a handful of conditions. It is pain in response to stimulus that would not normally elicit a pain response, but rather a touch, movement, or temperature sensation only. Consider the feeling of a severe sunburn, except that your skin doesn't look any different, and you know you have not had exposure to the sun. There's no redness or peeling, just extreme sensitivity. This can include pain from a simple touch (tactile allodynia), in which the fibro patient may find that at times it simply seems that his or her skin hurts to even the lightest touch. There can also be a response to something such as clothing or a breeze moving across the skin, known as mechanical allodynia. Another form, called thermal allodynia, may affect the way a fibro patient experiences temperature. Extreme hot or cold can cause a pain response in anyone, but fibro sufferers may find that heat or cold that is not extreme enough to normally be painful may still bring a pain response from the nerve endings in the skin.

> *I experience occasional allodynia, of any kind, but most often mechanical or tactile. There are times that just my husband rubbing lightly on my arm results in nearly unbearable pain. It can feel like scraping heavy coarse sandpaper- or a touch can feel like a needle or knife plunging into my skin and muscle. I experienced this for a year or so before I knew that it was from fibromyalgia.*

Other pain and muscle tissue-related symptoms associated with fibromyalgia can include stiffness and diffuse swelling and inflammation. These most often are at their worst when the fibromite first gets up in the morning. The joints and muscles often feel the way the average person would equate with the morning after having overdone a physical workout- except that this can happen daily for the fibromyalgia patient without having over-exerted at all. The diffuse (widespread/not localized) swelling can greatly contribute to the stiffness and soreness in the muscles and joints. Some fibro patients also notice swelling and puffiness in the lower extremities toward the end of the day.

Muscle twitches can also be present in fibromyalgia patients. These may range from conditions such as restless leg syndrome and other night-time spasms to around the clock muscle spasms in any part of the body, and anything in between. Many fibromites struggle with frequent "charley horses" and other painful muscle spasms. You will find other types of muscle spasms in the neurological symptoms section.

☺

My fellow fibromites may have felt a bit of humor, or at least a lightbulb of recognition at the description of the whole "voodoo doll" idea. That concept has been one I have seen used more frequently than any other by fibromyalgia patients to try and describe to the rest of the world how this condition feels. It isn't funny… not at all… but sometimes we have to laugh when others think of the idea as so foreign.

RESPIRATORY/SINUS SYMPTOMS

Another problem area for many fibromyalgia sufferers is that of respiratory or sinus-related symptoms. Many people have sinus or respiratory allergies, but there is a fairly high correlation between severe respiratory allergies and fibromyalgia- with 48% of fibro patients who also have severe respiratory allergies[11], versus 7-12% of the overall population[12]. The reasons for the correlation are unclear but it may be due simply to a higher sensitivity to allergens in the air such as mold spores and dust mites. Many fibromites also experience periods of unexplained shortness of breath (not from exertion), and it is thought this could be also related to the respiratory sensitivities to airborne particles.

There is also a higher rate of issues such as nosebleeds, pharyngitis (throat infection or irritation) and problems with the ears in those with fibromyalgia. The ear problems are generally not with hearing, but rather with itchiness and pain that would normally be associated with an ear infection- except that no infection is present. This makes treatment of this issue problematic since the primary and sometimes only treatment for ear infection pain and irritation is treatment of the infection itself, which treats the pain indirectly by resolving the underlying infection. It is clear to see, then, why this treatment would be completely ineffective in fibromyalgia ear pain, with no underlying infection.

SLEEP RELATED SYMPTOMS

In addition to the fatigue experienced as a symptom itself, most fibromites struggle with sleep difficulties up to and including extreme insomnia. This can take a few different forms, such as difficulty falling asleep, difficulty staying asleep, or poor quality of sleep. These difficulties often have nothing to do with how tired the person is or how much sleep they have had, or for that matter how much activity they have had. A fibromyalgia patient may only be able to sleep a few hours per night, despite being exhausted, or may sleep long hours but with little rest. A lack of REM[13] (Rapid Eye Movement) sleep may be largely to blame for both scenarios. Without deep sleep a person's body will not rejuvenate as well despite many hours of lighter sleep. In addition, staying in a lighter sleep can make it much easier for the patient to be awakened by minor stimuli. The cycle of deep sleep is part of what makes it easier to get back to sleep when we wake in the middle of the night, so if that cycle is lacking then the person may simply not be able to get back to sleep after a dog's barking wakes them up at 2:00 in the morning, for example.

> *Sleep tends to be one of my biggest struggles. I rarely sleep deeply enough to dream (which can sound like maybe a blessing) but the lack of REM sleep takes its toll. I also have difficulty getting to sleep, so that most days I'm only getting about 4 or 5 hours of non-REM sleep, with no REM sleep at all, and I wouldn't recommend it.*

Other culprits in the sleep disturbances of the fibro patient can include muscle spasms, such as restless leg syndrome, or other tremors which may worsen at night. Also the phenomenon known as "hypnic jerk"[14], or the falling sensation you sometimes get when first getting to sleep at night, can be made more pronounced by sleep deprivation or other sleep disturbances, and therefore can be a real problem for fibromyalgia patients, sometimes waking them several times each night. Fibromyalgia sufferers are also more prone to bruxism (grinding of teeth during sleep) in correlation with a tendency toward TMJD (Temporal-Mandibular Joint Dysfunction) syndrome, which causes problems in the joint and muscles of the jaw.[15]

REPRODUCTIVE SYMPTOMS

As much as we may not want to think or talk about this area of problems, the co-occurrence of reproductive system-related issues with fibromyalgia is such that this topic cannot be ignored. If you have experienced health issues connected with reproductive problems you are quite aware of how pervasive these can be. Even if your issue is not one of lack of ability to conceive, any issue involving the reproductive system can seem to take over your life at times.

In women with fibromyalgia (women make up 80-90% of fibromites[16]), the co-occurrence of issues such as fibroid tumors and other uterine and ovarian growths is not uncommon. These growths, though almost always benign, can come with other issues such as severe cramping and bleeding problems. With or without tumors or cysts, the co-occurrence of PMS/PMDD is extremely common, leading to abdominal and lower back cramping, among other issues. There is also a higher risk of miscarriage with any chronic health issue such as fibromyalgia, lupus, or chronic fatigue syndrome.[17]

This particular part of fibro is extremely frustrating, and can be heartbreaking. Due to fibroid tumors I have experienced extreme PMDD most of my adult life, which for me mostly consisted of searing pain and an abnormal cycle. I would do my best to keep a cheerful attitude, but at times it can be unbelievably challenging. I have also experienced 2 miscarriages- one due to the fibroids (miscarried at 6 weeks) and the other due to a chromosomal abnormality which took her from us in the middle of my second trimester. I have since had a hysterectomy due to the severity of the issues.

ABDOMINAL/ DIGESTIVE SYMPTOMS

Many fibromites also experience digestive symptoms, and IBS (irritable bowel syndrome) is another top associated co-occurring condition in those with fibromyalgia, with about 40% of fibro patients reporting such symptoms[18]. This is about double the occurrence in the general population[19]. With or without IBS, fibromites are often prone to nausea. In some nausea can be a common occurrence up to 4 or 5 days per week, spanning more than half of the day when it is present. The things that can exacerbate the nausea and/or IBS include certain foods, anxiety, visual or other sensory stimuli, lack of sleep, or electrolyte imbalance from dehydration, excessive salt, etc.

☺

What a fun subject, huh? I would like to formally apologize to anyone for whom the discussion of this particular subject gives rise to the symptoms discussed in this section!

COGNITIVE/ NEUROLOGICAL SYMPTOMS

Now to say that fibromyalgia comes with cognitive effects is not to say that fibromites are cognitively lacking. Many fibro patients feel that we have all of the 'brains' we did before we began experiencing fibro symptoms, but sometimes we simply cannot remember where we put them. Neurological symptoms can range from balance to concentration, and can have physical as well as mental and emotional repercussions.

Have you ever tried to remember something but you are feeling a bit fuzzy that day, so it's like you are trying to see through a thick fog? This is the type of mental sensation that is the root of the term "fibro-fog," coined by fibro patients and their doctors. If you can imagine that all of your mental abilities are still intact, but you just cannot get to them for some reason- as if they are just out of reach. The disorientation that accompanies this condition can be quite frightening. The National Fibromyalgia Research Association website describes it as well as any:

> ...it is one of the most life altering aspects of fibromyalgia. People who were accountants before fibromyalgia can [at times] no longer add up figures in their own checkbooks. Shopping center parking lots

become huge mazes with lost vehicles that a sick person in pain and with no energy must penetrate in order to get home.[20]

Some of the earmarks of fibro fog can include directional disorientation, or getting "turned around" (even in a familiar area), concentration difficulties, and memory impairment. The more common memory issue is with involuntary recall. In other words, the person doesn't have problems with remembering *how* to do things as much as remembering *to* do things. The problem we find is not that it is difficult to remember, it is simply so easy to forget!

Some of the physically manifesting neurological symptoms can include the paresthesias we touched on earlier and will discuss next, as well as balance and coordination issues. There are also types of neurologically based muscle twitches that, though not necessarily painful, can be irritating and downright scary. An example of this is the hand tremors that are often reported by fibromites. Though not documented officially as a symptom of or associated condition with fibromyalgia, these uncontrolled shaking twitches of the hand and arm muscles can be very disconcerting. Besides causing the patient to drop objects and have difficulty with everyday activities such as unlocking a door or writing legible notes, it is simply frightening to lose control of any part of your body.

The other medically defined type of pain, which we promised to address in this section, is known as painful paresthesia.[21] This is most easily understood as the type of "pins and needles" sensation most people have experienced at one time or another, which results from pressure on a superficial nerve. If you've ever had an arm, hand, leg, or foot "fall asleep," then you know the feeling. Now, imagine this feeling occurring quite regularly (daily in some patients) and imagine that it is not just tingly and unpleasant, but severe to the extent of being painful, every time. And imagine further that it is not caused by pressure or any other stimulus that can be distinguished, so there is no way to know how to avoid it happening daily, sometimes for several hours at a time. This is another phenomenon that is most common during the night time or in the early hours of the morning.

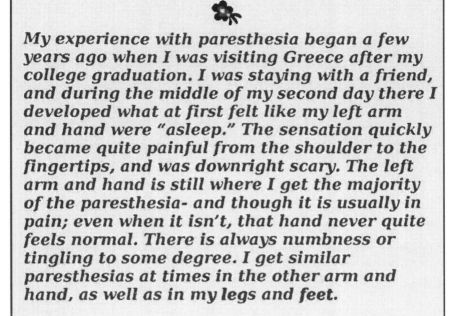

My experience with paresthesia began a few years ago when I was visiting Greece after my college graduation. I was staying with a friend, and during the middle of my second day there I developed what at first felt like my left arm and hand were "asleep." The sensation quickly became quite painful from the shoulder to the fingertips, and was downright scary. The left arm and hand is still where I get the majority of the paresthesia- and though it is usually in pain; even when it isn't, that hand never quite feels normal. There is always numbness or tingling to some degree. I get similar paresthesias at times in the other arm and hand, as well as in my legs and feet.

SENSORY SYMPTOMS

Fibromyalgia patients also experience increased sensitivity to several types of stimuli, as we touched on earlier with regard to headaches and sensory overload. In addition to heightened sensitivity to smell, sound, and visual stimuli, fibromites are often sensitive to barometric changes as well. Changes in the barometric pressure, temperature, and humidity can often trigger bodily pains and headaches in fibro patents. Because of this, weather changes can often bring about difficulty in getting around and conducting daily activities.

Earlier we touched on a sensitivity to light, sound, and smell which can worsen headaches and other physical issues in fibro patients. This sensitivity goes beyond just making an existing headache worse. Many fibromites actually find that there are times when their senses of hearing, sight, and smell seem to be more acute than others, so that noises sound louder, lights seem brighter, and smells seem stronger than they may to other people. It is this overstimulation of the senses that can cause a trip to any public place to be particularly exhausting.

The funny thing about this particular aspect is when a fibromite can smell a substance that most people can't. For me it is silk- I can smell silk if I come within about 20 yards or so. I can smell it when I am going through a department store that carries silk blouses or sweaters, or when I pass someone in the grocery store who is wearing it. I cannot wear silk because the smell drives me up a wall (it smells fishy, in case you were wondering).

EMOTIONAL SYMPTOMS

Fibromyalgia can also have an emotional impact.

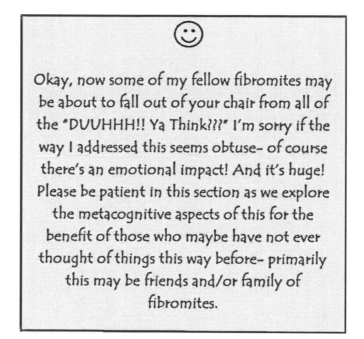

Okay, now some of my fellow fibromites may be about to fall out of your chair from all of the "DUUHHH!! Ya Think???" I'm sorry if the way I addressed this seems obtuse- of course there's an emotional impact! And it's huge! Please be patient in this section as we explore the metacognitive aspects of this for the benefit of those who maybe have not ever thought of things this way before- primarily this may be friends and/or family of fibromites.

It is not difficult to imagine that chronic widespread pain that can be triggered by almost anything would bring about some depression and difficulty dealing with life. In addition fibromites often may experience seemingly unexplained panic attacks and emotional withdrawal. It is not unusual for the patient to pull away from family and friends and seem to almost be a different person at times. The friendly outgoing personality may give way to one that is moody and introverted. The best thing family and friends can do is to maintain normality in the relationship as much as possible. Putting pressure or guilt on the fibro sufferer because of broken plans or what seems like a distant attitude during a time they are struggling with depression may cause them to pull farther away. Furthermore, if the people closest to the patient also pull away, the depression can deepen as the patient begins to feel guilt due to their own feelings about not being their usual cheerful self. As you can imagine, this can easily lead to a vicious cycle with regard to friend and family relationships.

There was a letter written by Ronald J. Waller which gives a great deal of understanding regarding the effects (largely the emotional effects) of fibromyalgia and does a wonderful job at painting the picture for those who don't know from first-hand experience what it can be like to deal with the day-to-day effects of fibro. The following quotes are excerpts from this letter, called "A Letter to Normals,"[22] that explain particularly well the emotional battle and the kinds of things many fibro sufferers would like to tell those around them.

> " You see, I suffer from a disease that you cannot see; a disease that there is no cure for and that keeps the medical community baffled at how to treat and battle this demon, who's[sic] attacks are relentless. My pain works

silently, stealing my joy and replacing it with tears. On the outside we look alike you and I; you won't see my scars as you would a person who, say, had suffered a car accident. You won't see my pain in the way you would a person undergoing chemo for cancer; however, my pain is just as real and just as debilitating. And in many ways my pain may be more destructive because people can't see it and do not understand...."

"Please don't get angry at my seemingly [sic] lack of interest in doing things; I punish myself enough, I assure you. My tears are shed many times when no one is around. My embarrassment is covered by a joke or laughter..."

"I have been called unreliable because I am forced to cancel plans I made at the last minute because the burning and pain in my legs or arms is so intense I cannot put my clothes on and I am left in my tears as I miss out on yet another activity I used to love and once participated in with enthusiasm."

"And just because I can do a thing one day, that doesn't mean I will be able to do the same thing the next day or next week. I may be able to take that walk after dinner on a warm July evening; the next day or even in the next hour I may not be able to walk to the fridge to get a cold drink because my muscles have begun to cramp and lock up or spasm uncontrollably. And there are those who say "But you did that yesterday!" "What is your problem today?" The hurt I experience at those words scars me so deeply that I have let my family down again; and still they don't understand...."

"On a brighter side I want you to know that I still have my sense of humor....I love you and want nothing more than to be a part of your life. And I have found that I can be a strong friend in many ways. Do you have a dream? I am your friend, your supporter and many times I will be the one to do the research for your latest project; many times I will be your biggest fan and the world will know how proud I am at your accomplishments and how honored I am to have you in my life."

"So you see, you and I are not that much different. I too have hopes, dreams, goals... and this demon.... Do you have an unseen demon that assaults you and no one else can see? Have you had to fight a fight that crushes you and brings you to your knees? I will be by your side, win or lose, I promise you that; I will be there in ways that I can. I will give all I can as I can, I promise you that. But I have to do this thing my way. Please understand that I am in such a fight myself and I know that I have little hope of a cure or effective treatments, at least right now. Please understand...."

SKIN/HAIR/NAIL RELATED SYMPTOMS

The primary skin and nail issues have to do with the tendency of the fibromyalgia patient toward tissue overgrowth. This produces pronounced ridges in the fingernails, ingrown hairs, lipomas (benign soft tumors), skin tags, and heavy cuticles that split painfully down into healthy skin tissue. The fibro patient also may experience mottled or ruddy skin, and a tendency to skin breakouts and allergies.

The primary hair related issue is the tendency for hair loss. The loss is temporary and is most pronounced during times of stress. Because the hair does not stop growing, the hair loss will most often not be severe enough to bring about baldness, but rather a sudden thinning.

I first experienced hair loss after a particularly stressful period a couple of years ago. Thankfully, I have a lot of hair, but noticed a great deal of hair in my brush and the drains. Then I started noticing that my hair was much thinner than usual. After doing a bit of research, I was surprised to find out that this is very common in fibro- especially during stressful times.

COPING WITH FIBROMYALGIA

We have taken a great deal of time and energy outlining what a fibromite goes through as a result of this condition, but to completely describe the problem without even touching on the solution- well that is just simply too depressing. There are ways to cope- not a cure, but things patients and their families can do to make the burden a little bit lighter.

One of the biggest weapons we have in this fight is attitude. Not just a positive attitude, but one of prayer and knowing that the Lord has us in His hand- and that not one challenge will confront us that *HE* does not have the strength to overcome, and that He will impart that strength to us as we need it. This is the most powerful tool in our arsenal.

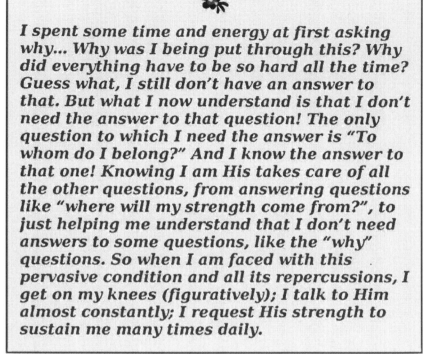

I spent some time and energy at first asking why... Why was I being put through this? Why did everything have to be so hard all the time? Guess what, I still don't have an answer to that. But what I now understand is that I don't need the answer to that question! The only question to which I need the answer is "To whom do I belong?" And I know the answer to that one! Knowing I am His takes care of all the other questions, from answering questions like "where will my strength come from?", to just helping me understand that I don't need answers to some questions, like the "why" questions. So when I am faced with this pervasive condition and all its repercussions, I get on my knees (figuratively); I talk to Him almost constantly; I request His strength to sustain me many times daily.

There are of course some other things, though none nearly as important as prayer, that the fibromite can do to help with this condition. Perhaps the one that seems like the biggest paradox is that of exercise. Although exertion, as we discussed, can leave the fibro patient feeling as if they have the flu- experts say that exercise can help to reduce the overall effect of the condition. The key, apparently, is in moderation and easing into a gentle exercise routine. Types of exercise highly recommended for fibromites are the gentle poses and movements of Tai Chi and Yoga. As you can imagine, I do not ascribe to the mystical elements of these activities, but I am working on implementing a daily routine of the physical movements and stretches.

Another way in which the fibromite can work to manage the condition is with diet. An important key to understanding how the diet can help is in understanding how fibromyalgia and hypoglycemia may actually go hand in hand.[23] Armed with this knowledge, a simple hypoglycemic diet is a good start. This diet is mostly a matter of avoiding simple carbohydrates (refined sugars and starches) and getting plenty of complex carbohydrates, fiber, lean protein, and of course drinking plenty of water (important in any diet). To find your minimum level of water intake, find your weight (in pounds) and divide by two. This is the *minimum* number of ounces of water you should drink every day.

The support of family and friends can be a big key for many fibromites, which is the whole point behind this guide. We deal with things more adeptly when we know we are not imagining things, and when we know we are not alone. If you or someone you love is dealing with this pervasive disorder, share this information with those around you. This is definitely an issue in which being informed makes all the difference.

STORIES

I have decided to include stories from the journeys of a few of my fellow fibromites. These only include, of course, information I have been given permission to include. The first is from a reader who has requested to remain anonymous.

This young lady is 35 years old and has noticed aches, pain, and generalized fatigue for years. It did not occur to her that fibro could be the reason until she saw a pulmonologist. This doctor did a palpation (pressing on various spots by hand) and after doing this exam and taking into account her history of extreme fatigue, he referred her to a rheumatologist. She had actually considered having both knee and ankle surgery for the pain she had been having. Possible diagnoses considered for her had included chronic fatigue and mononucleosis. She experiences sleep disturbances, dry eye, and dry mouth issues. Her fibro related issues are complicated by bipolar disorder and other accompanying medical conditions. These conditions pose a challenge to her doctors with respect to finding a medication combination that will be safe and effective in managing all of the health conditions, and as you can imagine necessitates all of her specialists communicating and working together to safely prescribe what she needs. When she was first diagnosed with fibro, she became very emotional and depressed. With help, she is getting some relief- and has found some relief in simply having a name to put to the condition. The ongoing battle with depression and sleep disturbances, as well as pain management, is one she is coping with on a daily basis.

LAURIE'S STORY

Laurie was diagnosed with the "Asian Flu" in January of 1981 at the age of 12. She was in bed for 3 weeks with fatigue, aches and pain, as well as fever. She believes it was actually mononucleosis, since last year she tested positive for Epstein Barr, the virus that causes mono. Within 2 years of her illness she began having unusual health problems. She began having skin issues, breaking out in hives from head to toe. She began having debilitating pain in her lower back, interfering with her physical activity. She was told she had scoliosis and that there was a vertebra missing in her lower spine.

After marrying in 1986, she had her first child in 1987, and had digestive problems during the pregnancy. The delivery was uncomplicated but soon after she was diagnosed with irritable bowel syndrome. The back problems also continued, and after seeing an orthopedist she was told she should never have any more children, and that the diagnosis for her back problems was actually rheumatoid arthritis. As you can imagine, when one is constantly given contradicting opinions, it becomes difficult to trust what has been said, so Laurie decided to ignore the orthopedist's advice. Her second child was born in 1994, and that pregnancy was similar to the first. After the birth, she experienced some improvement of her back pain, possibly a temporary remission.

Within a few years she began having problems with the reproductive organs, which prompted diagnoses of endometriosis, HPV virus, lesions, and stage 3 cervical cancer. The lesions were removed, and over the course of the next few years and many exams she was cleared of the cervical cancer diagnosis, and was also told the HPV was not present. With doctors again contradicting each other, this furthered her distrust of medical professionals.

In 2001 she had a bout with shingles, and in 2006 the endometriosis flared up again and she had surgery to burn away the uterine lining. This surgery is expected to stop the menstrual periods, but did not do so in Laurie's case. In 2009, the pain began to become more pronounced.

Laurie was slightly overweight, and with cholesterol and blood pressure that are naturally a bit high. She was told by her doctor that if she lost weight, the pain and all of the other health problems would subside. She began an exercise and weight loss regimen in 2010 and immediately began having bladder problems, and after only 8 weeks she broke her foot in what seemed like a minor fall. She had already lost 20 pounds at this point and had seen no improvement of her symptoms. Of course an injury of this type can inhibit weight loss efforts, but by this time Laurie had already begun to realize there must have been more than weight contributing to her health issues.

 She began researching all of her symptoms. At one point she thought she might have had multiple sclerosis, or that her problems were all related to the earlier diagnosis of rheumatoid arthritis. She kept seeing her doctor and was finally referred to a neurologist, who did tests and diagnosed her with fibromyalgia. She was also sent to a gynecologist who found excessive scar tissue on exam, and after ordering an ultrasound found that there were 4 tumors on the uterus and a bleeding cyst on one ovary. Due to family history and the severity of the problems, these findings led to a complete hysterectomy. Though this helped with some of the immediate issues with the endometriosis, it did not solve as much as she had hoped.

Many of the symptoms have since returned. She has also experienced costochondritis, and believed at the time that she was having a heart attack. She has also suffered a torn calf muscle after what seemed like it should have been a minor injury. She continues to suffer from skin breakouts, which make the hot summers where she lives extremely difficult. The soreness in her shoulders and neck is often accompanied by headaches.

Laurie tells me "Some of the strongest people I know suffer from this condition. My husband has watched me through all my problems and would argue that I am strongest person he knows. The problem is that the doctors I have dealt with (mainly Kaiser Permanente) want to [attribute]... my problems to stress, weight, being sexually abused (I have not been but I was told that everyone that has Fibromyalgia has been????), along with not having a high tolerance for pain (what?)."

Laurie says that outwardly she handles stress well, and has even been complimented on her ability to keep cool in stressful situations. She realizes that the problem is that her body then reacts physically to the stress. How does one control such a thing?

Laurie has maintained her weight loss, and though her cholesterol and blood pressure remain a challenge for her, she remains convinced the weight is not and was not the root of her health problems: "I know a lot of people who weigh more, are much larger and in poor health. They do not suffer the way that I do."

One of her primary concerns is that with this condition, she has had the problem of her muscles tearing easily. Without the ability to get regular, even gentle, exercise, she is concerned about how to address the issue. She has given up on help from doctors, understandable given her experiences. She wonders at the possibility of Epstein –Barr or some related virus being the root of the problem, but has had no success in finding a medical professional who will help her "connect the dots." She is thankful for her family, who are supportive as she continues her search for answers.

AMY'S STORY

Amy was officially diagnosed with fibromyalgia about two years after the symptoms began. She was in a great deal of pain, had noticed fatigue, and had experienced depression. She constantly felt exhausted, even after a full night's sleep. Her muscles were always terribly sore and her joints always stiff.

She had noticed the tendency of the pain to move around. One day her shoulders would hurt, and the next day the pain might be in her hips or legs.

She thought the issues might have been due to her being overweight, but even after losing a significant amount of weight, the pain and fatigue did not subside; in fact they got worse.

Amy is blessed with a good doctor who listens, but it seems that he still does not really understand her condition. She has tried many different medications, but none have been helpful yet.

She is now taking Cymbalta, and it seems to help some with the depression, but offers no relief from other symptoms. Amy has noticed work becoming even more difficult the last couple of years, with the exhaustion and difficulty with physical tasks.

Amy states that instead of feeling her thirty-four years as she should, she feels as if she is trapped in an eighty year old body. This is terribly frustrating, and though her family is loving and supportive, she senses their frustration as well.

CRYSTAL'S STORY

Crystal is a 26 year old woman who was diagnosed with fibromyalgia 2 years ago. This was after 7 years of searching for answers, with the interim including 4 surgeries and 7 different doctors, after which she finally learned of her diagnosis and found that her illness was not just in her head.

It started with pain in her right hand, for which she visited a doctor. The doctor ordered simple rest, which she followed. After weeks of rest, she was referred to a hand surgeon, who did an MRI and found nothing wrong. Knowing the pain in her hand was not her imagination, Crystal sought a second opinion. This doctor noticed small cysts in her hand and scheduled her for surgery. With 6 weeks of physical therapy after surgery the pain had still not subsided, and if anything was now worse. The doctor ordered more tests and an exploratory surgery. After 12 weeks in a cast and more than 10 more weeks of therapy, still there was no improvement. The doctor, clearly baffled, told her she needed yet another surgery to fuse the joint between the last row of carpal bones and the adjoining metacarpals, thinking this would eliminate the pain. She agreed out of desperation and had the surgery. After 12 more weeks in a cast and months of very painful therapy, this did bring her some relief, but pain and lack of healing caused by the plate in her hand caused enough problems that the plate had to be removed.

After moving to a new state and beginning a new job, the pain was still a problem, so she got a referral to a new hand surgeon near where she was now living. This doctor began asking other questions not seemingly related to the hand, and began looking for other medical conditions that would account for this pain with no evident visible problems. After running blood tests, this doctor diagnosed Crystal with lupus, and referred her to a rheumatologist.

This left her feeling lost, that after a blood test this doctor was telling her that everything she had gone through over the last few years may not have been necessary, or helpful at all. She went to see the rheumatologist, who said it was not lupus, with the numbers in her blood work being borderline normal. He told her that there was nothing wrong with her and that it was probably just depression, and that she should see a therapist. This appointment left her feeling even more lost, so after a call to the hand surgeon she was referred to a different rheumatologist. The second rheumatologist examined Crystal and told her the pain was all in her head, and accused her of making it all up. He referred her to a therapist and told her she needed antidepressants. Emotionally distraught and in pain she knew was real, she placed another call to her hand surgeon. Hoping to help her find a doctor who would help with this condition, the surgeon referred her to a top rheumatologist at UCLA. This trip involved a long drive, but was worth the trouble. Within 20 minutes of the beginning of the exam, this doctor diagnosed her with fibromyalgia. Using the test for tender spots and the medical history, the doctor had been able to find the answer that explained all of Crystal's conditions, and began her on prescriptions intended to help with the symptoms. The doctor gave her information and told her she could call if there were any questions before her next appointment.

After just a few weeks with the medical treatment and learning to deal differently with stress, Crystal began to notice some improvement in her pain. Now, 2 years later, she knows that the medications will not cure the condition, and has tried a few different meds looking for the best outcome, but she is learning to cope with the condition and is doing ok. She still has days of extreme pain, which is difficult for her family and friends to understand. She is also learning to deal with this, hoping that one day they will understand her condition.

Crystal sites how crazy it is when people compare fibromyalgia pain to other daily aches and pains and fatigue. She wants to try and make them understand that it is not just sometimes but always, and not just in the back but in both arms and legs too.

She wants them to understand that it's not just being tired, but that her head is so clouded that she can rarely think clearly. She just refers them to information that might help get the point across.

She has made up her mind not to be defined by her condition and will not let it run her life. She does her best to get up every day and try new things, but must listen to her body and know when not to push into new adventures. She knows that if it wasn't for the hand doctor's persistence in getting her in contact with a rheumatologist that would help, and if not for the rheumatologist that finally solved the mystery, she might still be just living with pain and believing doctors who told her it was all in her head. But now, thankfully, she has answers.

LYNNE'S STORY

I have decided to include Lynne's story in primarily her own words:

"Years ago, when I was young, I thought I was a normal child. How would I have ever known that my life would be turned upside down and forward backwards by the time I grew up?

So...what happens to your life when you have Fibromyalgia, well, you don't want it to define you, but can you really say it doesn't?

This is who I am, but later is what I became!

I love going into my barn, hearing the horses neighing as I arrive. The sweet smell of hay hanging in the air. Grabbing their brushes to clean off the morning shavings from their fine-tuned muscular bodies, smelling the aroma of each horse as I transform their beautiful bodies into shimmering coats of armor.

Best of all, picking up my western saddle, with the smell of leather and horse oils lingering together, and laying the saddle across my horse's back, getting her tacked up and ready for a trail ride.

Walking side by side, my horse and I would lazily drift out of the barn and into the drenching sunlight outdoors. I would lift my left leg up into the stirrup and easily pull myself up and swing my body over her back, feeling the warmth of the sun soaking into my clothes and my skin as my hands gently pick up the reins, feeling her powerful body of muscle adjust beneath me. We meld together and became one as we ride out towards the woods.

Off we go, her hooves plodding slowly on the sandy walkway, my body swaying in rhythm with hers, as we enter into the magical woods where everything comes alive. Her ears perk, listening for any sound that shouldn't be there, and always knowing, something is there before me. The sounds of crisp leaves crunching and churning under her hooves, the leather saddle creaking with our swaying movements and the soft leafy branches gliding across my arms making my senses come alive . The mingled smells of leather and horse, huge trees, mossy rocks, and dewy leaves are all so powerful and wonderful you can almost taste it. The sun slipping through the cracks of the leaves, splaying bouncing golden sun-rays across the ground and all over the rock walls. Sounds of trickling streams, splashing hooves, and birds everywhere, singing and flying, swooping and hunting, just enjoying their day. As I gaze upward, I see the beauty of the deep blue sky with its fluffy white clouds dancing all round us in its picture perfect way. What a peaceful ride this is, what a perfect day this is, I wish this day wouldn't end.

But....Fibromyalgia begins

Up until I was 11 years old, life seemed normal. I played outside all day in the nice weather with my friends on the farm, played hide and seek in the tall grass, but that was not to last. Strange things started happening from that time on and I developed severe allergies and slight asthma, then other odd symptoms started to sneak in. I started with sleep problems, in which I could not fall asleep, nor stay asleep, basically sleeping on and off all night and by morning I really didn't want to get up for school. If I thought that was bad enough, there was more to come, sleep paralysis was my next issue. At that time my mother didn't know what was wrong with me so she took me to see a doctor (our regular doctor was not available); this doctor was insulting, to say the least, and put me on tranquilizers for 3 months and said it is just my nerves. This would be the beginning of symptoms that I would not understand until now, at the age of 56. After taking the tranquilizers, the sleep paralysis did subside for a while. I will admit that my home situation with my father drinking every Saturday night didn't help my situation. I was not able to handle things as well as my two brothers, so I thought. As time went on I developed panic attacks around the age of 15. The first one appeared out of the blue while I was sitting watching a TV show with my mother and little brother; my father was out drinking. All of a sudden I started to feel dizzy, numb, tingly and a feeling of passing out came all over my body. I was shaking uncontrollably and my mom helped me onto the couch and called an ambulance. At the hospital, they were so nice. They explained to my mother that it was my nerves and they gave me a shot of something to calm me down. So, I had now become the nervous one in the family, as they called it back then. Seriously, nothing much was done about nervous problems in children, back when I was young. I had to deal with it myself...basically get over it!

As time went on, the sleep paralysis would come and go. I married at the age of 20 and had my first child at age 24 and my second at age 27. When I went into labor with my first child it was unbearable and they had to give me a lot of drugs, there were problems. After she was born I actually had drug withdrawals and while I was sleeping, flashbacks of being in labor and actually feeling the awful pain. I ached all over and my muscles were too weak to hold her to feed. I needed the support of a pillow to lay her against me so that I could hold her on my lap in the rocking chair to feed her. I didn't think this was unusual since I had such a bad delivery, so I never said a thing,

As my daughter was growing, I started with awful back pains. Creeping and crawling sensations were constantly going up and down my spine, with intense pain. I went to a Chiropractor, but the relief was for only a couple of hours. I just lived with it and had my second child. My son was an easy labor and I felt much better, however, my hips and back bothered me more than ever. I blamed the pain on having to carry my children and when they started to walk things did get better. Again, I thought this situation was normal. Of course, I had called my doctor about the hip and back pain and according to him, nothing was wrong.

As my kids grew I continually had problems with my nerves and started to have pains in the inside of my knees when I slept at night. My doctor, who didn't believe in anything, said just put a pillow between your knees when you sleep. So, I did and it did feel better, but as time went by more pillows would be added to relieve body pressure as I slept.

I was a stay at home mom at this point in my life and one day I didn't feel well, I felt sick to my stomach all day but it didn't develop into anything else, so I thought. A week later I became so tired I could barely stay awake. I went from not being able to sleep to sleeping all night, getting up in the morning, putting the kids on the bus, trying to do laundry, but going back to sleep, getting up to get the kids off the bus, lying back down to rest, making supper and getting the kids ready for bed and then back to bed. During this time I was shocked at how well I could sleep and sleep.

I made an appointment with my my physician because I thought I was anemic. Anemia runs in our family. When I arrived at his office I explained what was going on, so he took some blood work and then called and said I wasn't anemic, so that was the end of that, no explanation as to what it could be. I was just fine. So, for an entire year I lived by doing one thing at a time and then sleeping. Grocery shopping was the worst. I could barely make it back from the store without wanting to fall asleep while driving. Eventually, this sleepiness left me and life returned to normal and I never thought about it again, until later in my life.

As the kids grew, I went to work part time at my husband's family owned store. I started to notice that my back would pain me for no reason, then the bottom of my feet, my shins and the muscles in my toes would pull backwards in pain. Things kept moving around and I wasn't sure what was wrong, I only knew this wasn't normal. It would take me 3-4 steps to straighten out just getting out of my chair. Back to my doctors I went, and to my surprise he told me I was depressed! Hmmmm, I didn't feel depressed, I wanted to do everything, including walking my dogs, activities with my children, and I just had pain, nothing else! So...he put me on an antidepressant which made me sick to my stomach, so he gave me another, the same thing happened and then finally another. This one didn't make me sick to my stomach, but I watched TV all night long; I couldn't sleep. So, he gave me a tranquilizer to help me sleep. Now this was ridiculous! A drug to help me not be depressed and a tranquilizer to go to sleep, which only allowed me to sleep 2 hours. So, into the trash bucket the drugs went and life went on. No one at that time told me that anti depressants could help with nerve pain, so who knew? Plus, they didn't agree with me anyway.

Symptoms seemed to subside for a while and when my daughter was 12 years old and my husband and I bought a horse for her. My husband built everything for our horses, because they lived in our backyard. Our horses were breeding when we bought them, so we were limited in riding them that year. But I cleaned stalls, brushed them, took riding lessons, went trail riding, trailered our horses to friends houses to ride with them and took care of two foals when they were born the following year. My daughter was involved with 4-H and was showing her horse all over. It was a lot of work and I couldn't have enjoyed it more. I was still working part time, but things were okay, but not for long.

As time went by my daughter was going to college and I decided to go back, as well , to get my degree in accounting so that I could move on from the family business. It was at this time that things started to really turn. I was probably in my early 40's by now. My first college class was off campus at a satellite site. A few other people in my class, including myself, landed at the incorrect campus site. It was a cold night, and the campus site was not far away so we decided to walk. We ran/walked because it was cold, and ran/walked back to our cars at the end of the class.

The next day I went to work and when I went to walk down our stairs, my legs were in so much pain I thought I was going to fall. I was scared because this was not normal. I told my husband I needed to go home because I was going to fall down the stairs if I didn't. Things were now really starting to get strange. I started having trouble cleaning our horses stalls, my hip was really bothering me, so my husband and daughter started cleaning on some of my days, until finally I couldn't clean them at all. So...back to the doctor and he basically told me it was all in my head! End of story with this doctor. Unfortunately, it was the end of our horses being in my backyard. I could no longer take care of them so I ended up boarding them at a beautiful farm that my friends own. My horses love it there, but I wasn't able to see them much because they were an 1hr and 45 minutes away (one way)...too long a drive and I was in pain.

My mother, who was never sick a day in her life, came down with Lupus around the age of 60, so she asked me to see her Rheumatologist, and I did. Blood work showed an elevated sediment rate and she told me that my pain was NOT in my mind. However, at this point she didn't know what it was and I was to follow up with her in a few months. When I went back my sed rate was still elevated and she put me on a couple of medications, one was Celebrex and two others to try, if one or the other didn't work, whose names I cannot remember. Nonetheless, none of them worked. She decided to put me on Prednisone to rule out Fibromyalgia, and the Prednisone worked great. All of my pains subsided, but of course, you cannot stay on high doses of Prednisone, so when I was being decreased to 15 mg per day, the pain started to come back. By the time I was off the drug entirely, I was back in the same situation. She told me I did not have Fibromyalgia because i responded to the Prednisone. She decided to do an EMG and a muscle biopsy. The EMG came back normal. I kept calling her for months to set up the muscle biopsy because I wanted to get to the bottom of things, but she never returned my calls, so I decided to peruse a new doctor.

In August of 2004 I went to a large hospital in Boston MA and saw a new Rheumatologist. I now had started with dry eyes and my eyes were red, painfully dry and swollen, when I got up each morning, so a new symptom had arrived. It took hours to see him and when I got into his office, he asked me some questions, did a quick physical exam and put me on 5mg of Prednisone. He told me I could take this whenever I wanted to because it wouldn't hurt me and to take this other drug once a week and he would see me in three months. I was shocked because he didn't even order blood work. At home I began taking the prescribed medication; the prednisone helped, of course, but this other medication didn't do a thing. I thought it was an anti-inflammatory drug, so I decided to look it up on the internet, as I was only just starting to use the web at this point in time. To my shock, the drug was a cancer drug. This doctor never explained to me what I was taking, nor what each drug was being used for. I was angry that he didn't explain what he thought I had and what he felt would help and how the drugs worked. So..I left him to find another doctor.

At this point in my life I had been working full time for 3 years and just landed my dream job, so I wanted to continue to work, it was good for me.

I was given then name of a very good Rheumatologist down my way and to this day I do believe she is very good, but the problem was that each time I went for a visit I would see one of her assistants, not her, and each girl would have a different opinion on what I should be taking, which drug combination would be best to use. In the end, they wanted me to take weekly shots of methotrexate for the rest of my life(they didn't like the pill form because they said it didn't work as well). Well, I work! End of story, I cannot possibly take that much time out of work each week to get a shot, follow up with blood work, get to work and keep my job. In addition, I hadn't even talked to the doctor about it and they still didn't know what I had. They called it an unknown autoimmune arthritic condition...something very generic. So...on to a new doctor.

I was referred to a new Rheumatologist in Boston at Mass General Hospital. He is so very nice and understanding and works with me. By the time I got myself to him, I was in bad shape. I had burning in my knees, painful feet, aching all over, couldn't sleep from the pain, couldn't be touched on my skin, spinal pain, itching, shortness of breath, and everything else under the sun. Just all around sick, but I looked WELL as everyone with Fibromyalgia is told! My new doctor did so many blood tests trying to figure out what my medical issues were. At this point, I have Fibromyalgia, Sjogren's and Chronic Fatigue Syndrome. I say at this point, because anything can change. I asked him why I responded to Prednisone when the other Rheumatologist believes if you do respond you cannot have Fibromyalgia, and he explained that in studies, some people with Fibromyalgia do respond to Prednisone and other don't ,but it doesn't mean you do not have Fibromyalgia. He has prescribed many new and old medications for me to try, but no matter what I try the side effects are too much and I still want to work, even though work has become such a challenge every day. I know that my chances of working until I am 62 are pretty slim if I have to go on heavier medication to subdue the pain, but I am going to hang in there for as long as I can. I am taking a low dose of

Prednisone, with 6-8 Advils per day to keep my pain bearable. I
do believe his diagnosis of Fibromyalgia is correct. I have had all
of the pressure points at one time and at other times, hardly any,
I fluctuate. However, I wasn't sure about the Sjogren's but
looking back, he was right again. I actually started with dry
mouth and didn't realize it. I went from swallowing pills with
water, to milk, to applesauce, and not understanding why. My
saliva was slowly decreasing over the years and I hadn't realized
it. The Prednisone has helped keep my allergies under control,
because I can no longer take allergy shots. I react badly to them,
and the Allergy medications are too drying for the eyes, which
effects the Sjogren's. What a predicament!

I am seeing a Physical Therapist to help keep my muscles
moving and the pain down. A few months have passed and
physical therapy has helped. I will continue to see him to find
out how far I can push myself. Pushing too far will put me in a
Fibro flare and flat on my back with unbelievable pain. The most
I can hope for at this point in my life is to be able to walk my dog
again. I haven't been able to walk any distance in about a year
and I certainly cannot ride my horse anymore. I have lost that
joy and ability to Fibromyalgia. My muscles still continue to
cramp while walking, it is almost paralyzing. One day at work I
almost didn't make it to my car. My muscles went into spasms
that prevented me from walking. Finally after a few minutes, the
spasms subsided just long enough for me to make it to my car

before they started once more. Fibromyalgia is so unpredictable you never know when and how it will strike you down.

Today is a different day, after three months of physical therapy I have taken my dog for a walk to my mom's house and back. That is something I couldn't do many months ago. Unfortunately, I lost my mother on July 21, 2010. She had Lupus, Sjogren's, and Fibromyalgia, and she always said...but people think you look great and you can do everything! She was my best friend and the wisest mother one could ever have, she understood my situation fully and hopes that I do not develop Lupus along with everything else. My story is genetically linked to my mother. It is well known that children of mothers with Lupus and Fibromyalgia have a greater chance of having Fibromyalgia and Sjogren's, but no one knows how things will progress. I haven't been diagnosed with any Lupus and hope not to be. Everyone is different, people need to respect that! This is a very misunderstood disease.

For now, my journey ends here. I will tell you that who I was before is not who I've become now....Fibromyalgia has changed my life, but I refuse to be defined by my Fibromyalgia. I was blessed, as so many people with Fibromyalgia were not, to have had many good life experiences before hitting the more challenging parts of living my life with Fibromyalgia. I have more compassion for people who have challenges in their lives that they cannot control and I believe that people can look well and be sick. In our society and medical communities today, people with Fibromyalgia need to be treated with respect and compassion. Who knows where it will strike, let us hope the non-believers don't have to find out!

ESTA'S STORY

Esta has a website all about fibromyalgia, which can be found at http://fibromyalgia-facts-fictions.com/index.html. Her story begins with a statement that she has had difficulties in getting doctors to understand and believe what she is telling them, and with them telling her it is all in her head. Unfortunately, as we have seen, this is all too common.

For Esta's story I will include quotes, or near-quotes, directly from her story's page on her website:

"Dealing with a person with a chronic sleep disorder

We have some long standing social mores that say if you are still in bed when everybody else is up, you must be lazy, no matter that you have good reason for it. But, unlike others with an accepted aliment, most people don't think that we with FM have good reasons.

This leads to comments of "Hey lazy bones" or other sarcasm, when you get up at noon or later from family, friends and the world at large. Never mind the fact you got to sleep at dawn.

One of the main reasons for this is that most people seem to think (as well as most doctors) that all you have to do is get your bio rhythms turned back around and everything would be just dandy. It does not matter how much proof there is to the contrary, the refrain is always the same... if you would just......

As that's how it is... for most people. Insomnia is a temporary state, like jet lag, that is curable. Heck, you can buy meds for it over the counter; that's how simple most people tend to think occasional insomnia is. This is not the case for those with FM.

No amount of making yourself go to bed at 10 PM every night and force yourself up at 7 am, to "establish" a sleep pattern is going to help a bit, other than to increase pain.

I know; I've done it, repeatedly. Sleeping pills only work for short periods of time, and even with that enforced sleep, the body goes right back to "Up all night" the second the meds are withdrawn. Insomnia for us is chronic, as the neurochemistry that allows one TO sleep, has been seriously disrupted.

No person with FM chooses this state of affairs; it's something that happens to them, like a train wreck, every night of their life. I cannot count the number of nights I have lain in bed and begged for rest, just one night of decent, unbroken, restful sleep.

As all it takes is the dog barking, a train whistle, turn over in your sleep and the pain of your joints jolts you out of your doze and you're awake again, for another hour or so, finally fall back asleep, only to be jolted out again. This happens over and over. You spend your nights tossing like a top, in pain, up and down like a yo-yo, until your eyes are so tired they are weeping and blurred.

The last thing I want to hear, when I drag my still tired, stiff and aching body outta bed, after I finally passed out for a few hours, is "Good morning lazy bones" . This is beyond uncalled for.

A small peek into almost every morning of my life

You crack open your eyes and the first thing you notice when you try and move is that you hurt. Most of the time, since your body's homeostasis is shot, you have spent that last hour before you awake sweating, no matter what the temperature is in the air. Which means your body is now damp and cold. So you wake up and now you're chilled, which kicks off all the joints into pain. Since your muscles have not moved in sleep, the MPS and FM points will flare into pain, the moment you try and move.

The first move of the day can [rather WILL] mean a wince, to an outright cry out in pain, and since you're chilled too, you're shivering. So you try and sit up, now your stomach, which has been merrily building up acid all night, kicks in the second you try this, often to the point where it forces you to lay right back down because of the acid reflux.

Not to mention, that to sit up too fast will make you literally dizzy. So you sit up in stages, otherwise you are liable to throw up. Half an hour or so later of sitting up in stages, you are now sitting up, huddled into your blankets, because you are still cold.

Now you have several choices: you can go and get a hot shower, which will help, but such action has its own problems, as it means you have to bend and stoop to undress, climb over the tub rail to get in, raise your hands to wash your hair, lower the body to wash your feet; Which you avoid doing as you are so nauseous at this point that to lean over means you feel like you're about to throw up. And occasionally, you do. There's nothing in your stomach but acid, so you get a badly burned throat and nasal passages when this happens.

Ladies, any of you who have had children recognize this state, it's called morning sickness. Now picture that every morning of your life and you have a good idea of what a person with FM lives with.

If you opt for the shower you have to dry off quickly, or get chilled again, so that by the time you finish drying off you are panting and out of breath. But now you have to dry your hair, as you do not dare run around with a wet head, as you will just get chilled again if you do. This trashes any benefit your arms, shoulders, neck may have gotten from the warm water.

Most days you just skip the shower [until later], as to do so means you have to rest by the time you're done. You just bundle up until you are warm.

 No matter if you take the shower or not, you now jump right back into the thermal underwear you were wearing when you went to bed, unless it's summer, as you're almost always cold [or some of us have right the opposite problem]. You make sure you have on socks and might even put on a hat to keep body heat.

So now you toddle off to the kitchen, since you have just sweated off a good deal of water, you're very thirsty. You don't even think about eating. The very idea of food makes you blanch, so you don't even consider it. You notice the smells in the kitchen, which makes you even more nauseous.

By the time you get your drink you are tired and need to rest; you are literally breathing hard. But you know you need to move so you lightly stretch and try and work out all the muscles. By the time you do that, now you really have to sit down, and all of this is due to just the act of GETTING UP !

You finally give up on the idea of the acid, which is not going away, and either drink some of the liquid chalk you find in most antacid bottles or chew up a few dry tablets in lieu of any food. Then you get to spend the next hour or so belching, as excess gas is about half of your stomach's trouble. Your mouth feels like you have been chewing on pennies all night, with a coppery taste that never really goes away.

Welcome to my morning :)

Now just to top it off, a really short look into my day after all that

Now, on to your day- for me it means in front of the computer, as that's my job now since I had to give up other trades. By the time I sit down in front of it however, my arms and shoulders already hurt and my hands don't work well. I am trying hard to ignore the fire that's in my stomach and just pay attention to what's in front of me.

It can take me the better part of several hours just to answer my email. Why? Because anything they require me to do, generally I do right now so I don't forget about it, since the short term memory is gone. Meaning for me, anything a client needs gets done *right now*. Updates to pages, change this, add that, make this image etc. has to get done, right after I read the email.

Unless it's more than I can handle at that moment, in which case it has to go on my little pop up and bug me reminder program. And if I do not put on that program they may as well have not asked me, as it went past my eyes and right past the brain. So I save all letters and hope that I remember them.

Now all of this is lots and lots of repetitive moves by the hands. The hands I have to stop and massage every half hour. The ones that if I don't do that, just flat stop responding. I tell them type and the hand sits there, to where I have to deliberately think about moving the fingers. After a few hours of this, I am really tired now, my hands are numb, my shoulders hurt, my eyes are blurred, my back and legs ache, I normally have a headache.

My tail bone is all but rubbed raw from how often I have to lean into the screen in order to see clearly or shift position due to the body's pains. Despite all you try to do, the bio mechanics of how you sit etc. is decided by your body's demands, not what you know to be good posture.

You fight a forever war with the body of what is "good posturing" versus the odd and contorted positions in which you find yourself as the body is trying, HARD, to avoid more pain, so it literally twists and contorts you which causes more pain for the other muscles that wind up under stress.

I court bed sores, yes you heard that right, or "pressure sores" as they are more properly called on the tail bone, elbows and heels on a regular basis on account of this. As they take a great deal of pressure just to move the body about. Ask anyone who is wheel chair bound and they can tell you all about it.

You tend to use the elbows to move the body, as the legs no longer work right. It hurts too much to use them to shift the body, so like our paraplegic cousins, you drag the body's weight on the elbows. The tail bone is particularly vulnerable, because you have to have your legs up when seated, which means that your entire body weight is centered on a very small part of your anatomy, and it protests this treatment rather loudly. The right chair cushion becomes a serious consideration."

"By the time I reach this point, I have to get up and go lay down a while, read a book maybe. I might even nap if I am lucky and come back to it a few hours later ... maybe. As the labor I just did might well be all I'm good for- for the day.

So a few hours of work just might take me all day to do, for all the breaks I have to take in order to accomplish it at all. And this is assuming mind you, that I don't have an IBS attack going, or a whole host of other possible energy drains; as if so, cut the workability down more for every other issue I might have going on.

Understand now, and make note: I have yet to eat, so I am doing all this on no fuel whatsoever. Nor will there be any until much later in the day, when the stomach etc., settles down and allows me to eat."

"You PAY dearly for anytime you have a good day and over-do it. (which we ALL do. The good days don't come often and you try and get all the things done that you had to let slide.) Then often go down for a week or more of pain, paying for that indiscretion. "Push and Crash" it's called.

You make deals with yourself regarding the housework and any other responsibilities.

You, who could once take care of yourself and anybody else who came along.

Now we have to choose if we are going to do dishes today, or do the rug, because often we can't do both. Energy is finite and has to be rationed out carefully, or there will be none left for the 'Gotta Do' things"

"My eyeglass script has changed 6 times in less than 9 years due to MPS (myofacial pain trigger points) interfering with the ocular muscles.

They tried to give me bifocals. I can't wear them. Why? Because, looking down hurts, just like looking up or sideways. To look in my side mirrors in the car I have to turn the whole head, which also hurts, but less than trying to move my eyes.

Also, there are the hands that go numb from using the mouse, holding a book, picking up a grandchild.

Vacuuming the rug can mean spending the rest of the afternoon cuddled up with a heating pad, for hands, shoulders, back. (that same heating pad that lives in your chair... forever)

I can't lay down to sleep but have to be propped up in an EZ chair (a night in a flat bed is a promise of worse pain, so much so, that to get out of that bed you'd need help). An adjustable bed might help, but they are far too costly for someone who is unemployed, and no medical coverage will pay for one for our condition."

"To get a hug from someone can sometimes mean having to grit your teeth so that they don't notice they just hurt you doing it. You learn not to shake hands, or let anyone hug you on most days, as it's painful. This isolates you. Some days just to touch you, even lightly, is too much.

You see, what is an 'ow' to normals, for those with FM can be 'OWWWWWWWW!' due to excess substance P, a pain receptor in the spine and due to changed nerve endings. This hypersensitivity extends to other things as well.

You are extremely sensitive to things like certain sounds for example, as the body interprets the onslaught of noise as painful. A fact I only recently learned."

Esta's experiences tell her that if she had known more about this condition earlier:

"I would have been better armed to deal with my doctors; I would not have spent years of self-recrimination thinking I was what my doctors, and often my mates, said I was: that I was just a hypochondriac who was looking for attention, with all the hospital trips for migraines, with the upset stomach after dinner, and a million other things that, taken one at a time, meant little and don't add up to anything; but all together mean a whole lot, and it has a name...which was a glorious thing to hear, because it meant that I was NOT imaging it.

I was NOT a whiner, who just wanted people to feel sorry for me.

I was ... near to the point of believing that crap. The fact that I felt just as bad, no matter if anyone was around to see me or not, didn't seem to matter to anyone but me, and I gave up even trying to explain that.

That I was NOT gonna die from how bad I felt... what a burden that lifted ... but I know what is wrong and can work on helping myself."

"That is what knowing that this feeling had a name gave me, hope... that someday someone would figure out why and be able to cure it, or at least make a better quality to life, and in the meantime I do all that I can to make life survivable, and sometimes even joyful."

MOVING FORWARD

I hope that this book has helped in the understanding of friends and loved ones, as well as fibromites, as to exactly what we are up against. Although all of our stories are different, the one constant is hope- the hope for effective treatments, or even a cure; the hope for understanding among those who walk by our sides. So, Fibro Fighters... share this information... keep up hope... and remember to whom you belong!

EPILOGUE

I would like to offer a special word of thanks to my fellow fibro
fighters who contributed their stories and offered their
encouragement for this project. I also am very grateful to my
family: I have a wonderful supportive husband, Curtis Bolton; an
amazing son who inspires me every day, Isaac Bernardo; a loving
and encouraging mother, Lauren Vines Taite, and grandmother,
Pauline Zacharevitz, who have both given me a wonderful
example and helped with editing, and more support and love
from the rest of my family and church family at First Community
Church in Crandall, TX, than I ever could have hoped for.

I'd also like to thank those working so hard to raise awareness of
this debilitating disorder. If you'd like to help in this quest, visit
THUNDERSTRUCK! at http://fibromodem.com/?p=9614.

Author's Recommended Resources:

Don't forget, fibromyalgia awareness day is May 12 of each year. Watch http://www.fmcpaware.org for more information.

To ask questions of medical experts, try the forum at http://exchanges.webmd.com/fibromyalgia-exchange .

For in-depth articles about various aspects of fibromyalgia, check out http://www.mayoclinic.com/health/fibromyalgia/DS00079/TAB=indepth

Find information, articles, and a discussion community at http://www.fibromyalgia.com/

Other forums:
http://fibromyalgia.forumotion.com/
http://www.dailystrength.org/c/Fibromyalgia/forum
http://www.fibromyalgiaforums.org/

Online fibromyalgia tests and questionnaires can be found at:
http://www.fibromyalgia-information-relief.com/fibromyalgia-test.html
http://arthritis.about.com/od/fibromyalgia/l/blfibroquiz.htm

Other information sites:

http://www.myalgia.com/

http://www.uptodate.com/contents/fibromyalgia-beyond-the-basics

http://www.ncbi.nlm.nih.gov/pubmedhealth/PMH0001463/

Make Donations for Fibromyalgia Research:

http://www.afsafund.org

(a percentage of all proceeds from sale of this book will be donated to fibromyalgia research)

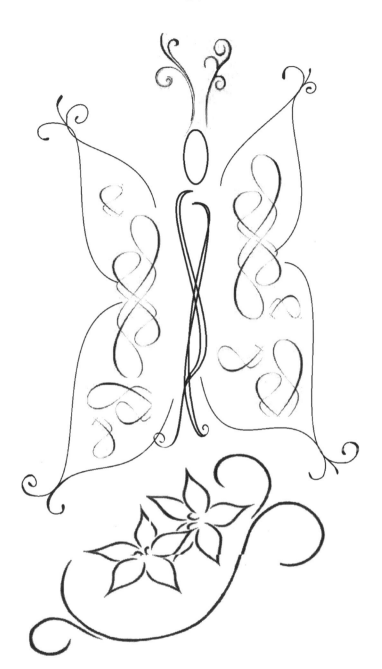

FIBROMYALGIA JOURNAL:
Tell your own fibro story!

_____

_____

_____

_____

_____

_____

_____

_____

_____

_____

_____

_____

_____

_____

_____

_____

_____

_____

_____

_____

SOURCES

1

http://www.businessweek.com/lifestyle/content/healthday/64
1874.html;
http://www.fmaware.org/site/PageServer?pagename=fibromya
lgia_science
2

http://www.fmaware.org/site/PageServer?pagename=fibromya
lgia_diagnosed

3 http://www.nfra.net/Diagnost.htm

4 Clark, R.K. (2005). *Anatomy and physiology: understanding the human body*. Jones and Bartlett Publishers, Inc.

5 Ostalecki, S. (2008). *Fibromyalgia: The Complete Guide from Medical Experts and Patients.* Jones and Bartlett Publishers.

6 Shomon, M. (2004). *Living well with chronic fatigue syndrome*. New York, NY: HarperCollins Publishers, Inc.

7 Matallana, L. (2009). *The complete idiot's guide to fibromyalgia*. Penguin Group, Inc.

8 From "Understanding Fibromyalgia Pain,"
http://chronicfatigue.about.com/od/whatisfibromyalgia/a/fibr
omyalgiapain.htm
9 http://www.fibromyalgia-
symptoms.org/fibromyalgia_chest_symptoms.html

[10] http://painresearch.utah.edu/crc/CRCpage/terms.html

[11] http://www.nutramed.com/fibromyalgia/fmdef.htm

[12] Pleis, JR, Ward, BW, & Lucas, JW. U.S. Center for Disease Control, National Center for Health Statistics. (2010). *National health interview survey* (Vital Health Stat. (10)249). Washington DC: US Government Printing Office.
[13] http://www.webmd.com/sleep-disorders/excessive-sleepiness-10/sleep-101

[14] http://www.sleepdisordersguide.com/topics/hypnic-jerk.html

[15] http://www.fibromyalgia-symptoms.org/fibromyalgia_tempero.html

[16] http://www.fibromyalgia-symptoms.org/fibromyalgia-statistics.html

[17] Wilson, R. (2004). *Recurrent miscarriage and pre-eclampsia.* Hackensack, NJ: World Scientific Publishing Co. Pte. Ltd.

[18] Marcus, D, & Deodhar, A. (2011). *Fibromyalgia: a practical clinical guide.* New York, NY: Springer.

[19] http://digestive.niddk.nih.gov/ddiseases/pubs/ibs/

[20] http://www.nfra.net/fibromyalgia-fibro-fog.htm

[21] See footnote [8] on page 8.

[22] http://www.depressionforums.org/forums/topic/29447-fibromyalgia-a-letter-to-normals/

[23] Marek, C. (2003). *The first year: fibromyalgia.* Marlowe & Company. p#169.

Printed in Germany
by Amazon Distribution
GmbH, Leipzig

16280297R00059